Diabetes & Pregnancy:
What to Expect

Fourth Edition

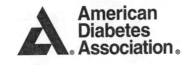

American
Diabetes
Association®

Director, Book Publishing: John Fedor
Associate Director, Consumer Book Acquisitions: Sherrye Landrum
Editor: Janet Cave
Production Manager: Peggy M. Rote
Composition: Circle Graphics, Inc.
Cover Design: Wickham & Associates, Inc.
Printer: Port City Press, Inc.

Printed in the United States of America
1 3 5 7 9 10 8 6 4 2

The suggestions and information contained in this publication are generally consistent with the *Clinical Practice Recommendations* and other policies of the American Diabetes Association, but they do not represent the policy or position of the Association or any of its boards or committees. Reasonable steps have been taken to ensure the accuracy of the information presented. However, the American Diabetes Association cannot ensure the safety or efficacy of any product or service described in this publication. Individuals are advised to consult a physician or other appropriate health care professional before undertaking any diet or exercise program or taking any medication referred to in this publication. Professionals must use and apply their own professional judgment, experience, and training and should not rely solely on the information contained in this publication before prescribing any diet, exercise, or medication. The American Diabetes Association—its officers, directors, employees, volunteers, and members—assumes no responsibility or liability for personal or other injury, loss, or damage that may result from the suggestions or information in this publication.

∞ The paper in this publication meets the requirements of the ANSI Standard Z39.48-1992 (permanence of paper).

ADA titles may be purchased for business or promotional use or for special sales. For information, please write to Lee Romano Sequeira, Special Sales & Promotions, at the address below.

American Diabetes Association
1701 North Beauregard Street
Alexandria, Virginia 22311

Library of Congress Cataloging-in-Publication Data

Diabetes & pregnancy : what to expect.
    p. cm.
    Includes index.
    ISBN 1-58040-071-X (pbk. : alk. paper)
    1. Diabetes in pregnancy—Popular works. I. Title: 4th ed. II. American Diabetes Association.
RG580.D5 T37 2001
618.3—dc21

RG580
.D5
T37
2000

00-066394

Table of Contents

Acknowledgments

This book was produced and written by members of the Task Force for the American Diabetes Association Council on Pregnancy. These members include: Lois Jovanovic, MD, Chair; Nancy Cooper, RD; Marion Franz, RD; Priscilla Hollander, MD; Donald Coustan, MD; Robert Emling, MS, EdD; Lisa M. Fields, RN, MSN; Robin Goland, MD; John Hare, MD; Ronald Kalkhoff, MD; Deborah McCoy, RN, MS; and Candace Wason, RN, MS.

We thank the reviewers for their time and expertise, including Pasquale J. Palumbo, MD; Steven G. Gabbe, MD; and Kathleen Wishner, PhD, MD.

We heartily thank Lois Jovanovic, MD, for her review and revision of the second, third, and fourth editions. We also thank Carolyn Leontos, RD, CDE, MS, and Deborah McCoy, RN, MS, for their review of the third edition, and Carol Homko, RN, CDE, MS, for her review of the fourth edition.

Section 1

Introduction

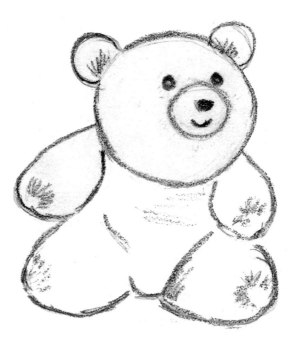

Deciding to have a baby is one of the great decisions of your life. That one decision will result in numerous changes for at least the next 20 years: rattles, teddy bears, diapers, a crib; scuffed-up knees, toys in the driveway, kindergarten, back-to-school sales, school plays, the PTA; requests for the car, your permission, your approval, your wallet; college funds, fraternities, sororities, graduation parties; and more joy than you can imagine right now.

But, before all this takes place, you have to make the decision to do what it takes to give birth to a healthy, happy baby. And reading this book is the first step in making that decision.

♥ Chapter 1

Diabetes, Pregnancy, and You

You're reading this book because you're thinking about having a baby and you want to know more. It is true that, in the past, pregnancy did present major problems for women with diabetes. But that's not the case today for most women.

Before insulin was introduced, women with diabetes rarely became pregnant, and if they did, their babies did not often survive. When insulin became available in the early 1920s, pregnancies became more common. Still, the number of successful pregnancies remained far below that of women who did not have diabetes.

The good news is that we now know that the key to a successful pregnancy for a woman with diabetes is tight blood glucose control both before conception and throughout pregnancy. Tight blood glucose control means achieving a normal blood sugar (glucose) level by checking blood glucose several times a day and balancing meals, exercise, and insulin. The goal of tight control is to keep blood glucose levels as close to nondiabetic or "normal" as possible. With tight control and good obstetrical care, today the chances of having a successful pregnancy are almost the same as for a woman without diabetes. (Obstetrics is the medical specialty that deals with childbirth.)

Although the rate of successful pregnancies among women with diabetes has greatly improved, there are still some problems with which we need to be concerned. One problem is that the rate of birth defects in children born to women who have diabetes remains higher than among those born to nondiabetic women. Approximately 2 out of 100 normal (nondiabetic) pregnancies will result in babies with birth defects. For women who have diabetes, the range of birth defects is 2 to 23% and is dependent on the level of a woman's glucose control at the start of the pregnancy.

Fortunately, however, we are learning how to increase the odds of producing healthy babies among women who have diabetes. We now know that many birth defects are related to the mother's blood glucose control before conception and during the first eight weeks of pregnancy. This is because it is during this critical time that the baby's organs are formed. One problem is that many women may not even know they are pregnant during this time.

The solution to the problem is obvious: You must plan ahead for your pregnancy. If you don't already practice good diabetes control regularly, that should be your first priority before you think further about having a baby. We suggest that a woman try to maintain good blood glucose control for three to six months before she plans to become pregnant. (Of course, good control should be a lifelong practice.) The HbA_{1c} test shows how well you are achieving good control. Your aim is an HbA_{1c} level close to 6% before you try to get pregnant.

It Takes Commitment

There has never been a better time for you, as a woman with diabetes, to plan for a pregnancy. By following a prescribed diabetes treatment program, you have a much better chance of giving birth to a healthy baby. But you will need to be committed to the work that pregnancy will take. It will certainly help if your partner is committed as well. This commitment should be based on a complete understanding of what is needed to achieve your goal. The fact that you're reading this book shows that you want to know more and that you care about your health and the health of your baby.

You will need and want a program of care that will help you obtain good blood glucose control and will allow careful monitoring of your baby's progress. This program will require regular visits with your obstetrician and other members of your health care team. The program will also include a variety of laboratory tests. It is possible that you might even be hospitalized for a time during your pregnancy, but only if problems arise.

Finally, care for women with diabetes during pregnancy is highly specialized. For this reason, you need a health care team on your side. What is a health care team? It is a group of health care professionals who specialize in the different aspects of diabetes care. Your team could include the following:

- a **physician** or **endocrinologist** who specializes in diabetes care and who is familiar with managing diabetes during pregnancy
- an **obstetrician** who specializes in high-risk pregnancies and is experienced in managing pregnancies of women who have diabetes
- a **pediatrician** or **neonatologist** who knows and can treat the special problems that can occur in a baby born of a woman who has diabetes
- a **diabetes nurse-practitioner** who can advise and teach you how to manage your diabetes
- a **registered dietitian** who can adjust your meal plan to meet the needs you will have during your pregnancy

Even with the help of these health care professionals, following a good diabetes program during pregnancy won't be easy. It will take a lot of time and can sometimes be frustrating. It can also be expensive. However, all this time, energy, and effort can make all the difference in the health of your baby.

This book is designed to provide the information you as a woman with type 1 diabetes need to have a successful pregnancy. (Editor's note: This book is specifically for the woman who has type 1 diabetes or type 2 diabetes that is controlled by taking insulin.

How does the team approach work?

Controlling diabetes is not always easy—even under the best of circumstances. It takes time and commitment to be responsible for your own health. Fortunately, you don't have to do it all alone. The American Diabetes Association (ADA) recommends you use the health care system to its fullest through the "team approach" to diabetes care. A health care team consists of experts in different aspects of health care in general, and diabetes care in particular.

Each person's health care team should meet his or her very personal health care needs. Therefore, your team may include different health care practitioners during different times in your life. Pregnancy is one such time.

The team approach helps your doctor provide you with expert care for all your specific needs. Diabetes care teams often include:

- a **diabetologist** or **endocrinologist** who specializes in diabetes care and treatment. This person usually heads the team.
- a **nurse-practitioner, nurse-clinician,** or **nurse-educator**. This is a registered nurse who works with your physician to provide you with diabetes care. These nurses usually are trained to instruct and advise you about managing your diabetes. Often, it is this individual you will talk to on the phone for routine management decisions or special sick day procedures. You may check in with this member of your health care team more often than the others.
- an **obstetrician** who specializes in high-risk pregnancies and is experienced in managing pregnancies of women who have diabetes. This health care professional is familiar with the extent of care that women with diabetes require when they become pregnant.
- a **registered dietitian (RD).** This person can help you design meal plans that meet your body's unique nutritional needs. As you grow older and your lifestyle and medical needs change, your diet will change as well. Your RD will help you tailor your meal plans to reflect those changes.

- an **eye doctor.** This person can monitor the condition of your eyes and watch for eye disorders that are common among people who have diabetes, such as retinopathy. **The ADA recommends an eye examination when you decide to become pregnant and again when you become pregnant. If you do have diabetic retinopathy, frequent eye exams are necessary throughout pregnancy.**
- a **social worker** or **psychologist.** This person can help you and your family members cope with any stress or anxieties that may come from learning to adjust to the diabetes lifestyle. These professionals can help you devise strategies for better relationships and teach you ways to reduce stress.
- a **podiatrist.** This health care professional is trained to give proper care to your feet. Proper daily footcare is important for people with diabetes and should never be overlooked.
- a **dentist. The ADA recommends that you have regular dental checkups.**
- **you,** the individual with diabetes. You are the most important member of the health care team because you call the shots. Like a quarterback on a football team, you must keep in touch with your health care team to let them know how you are doing and whether you need help.

If you don't have a health care team, your doctor may be a good source to help you find other health care practitioners to meet your specific needs. ADA may also be able to help. Many hospitals also have listings of health care professionals.

The team approach was developed for people with diabetes. It recognizes that people with diabetes are not sick; but rather, that people with diabetes require special guidance in maintaining their health.

Do not hesitate to contact your health care practitioners when you have questions. Remember, they are there to help you.

How Your Baby Develops

During the nine months that you are pregnant, a lot of changes will take place. The end result of that pregnancy will change your life forever—you'll be a mother and responsible for the care of another human being. It's exciting and a big responsibility—one that really begins before you become pregnant. In fact, it's possible that the most important care you ever give your child will be in those first few weeks of your pregnancy—a crucial time for the development of your baby.

Of course, each stage of your baby's development before he or she is born is important. And the best way to take care of your baby during this time is to take good care of yourself. If you are healthy, chances are good that your baby will be healthy, too.

Still, problems can occur. Finding problems and correcting them early are also important to the health of your baby. Numerous tests are available to help monitor and improve the success of your pregnancy. That's why regular checkups with your health care team are so important during each month of your pregnancy. You may need to have appointments with your health care team every two weeks in the last trimester of your pregnancy, and increase to once a week in the last month.

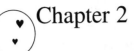

Chapter 2

What to Expect in the Nine Months

A normal pregnancy lasts 40 weeks, which is about 10 lunar months (4 weeks each) or 9 solar months (4 1/3 weeks each). Pregnancy—technically known as gestation—is broken down into 3 three-month periods called *trimesters.* Each stage is exciting as your baby develops and acquires all the physical characteristics he or she needs to live outside the womb. To give you an idea of your baby's progress, we will describe the different stages of development that normally occur during each trimester.

The first trimester In the first few weeks, your baby's heart forms and begins pumping blood. The digestive system, backbone, spinal cord, and brain begin to form. The placenta also develops during the first trimester. The placenta is the organ that provides needed hormones to keep you, your pregnancy, and your baby healthy. It provides a filtering system to allow the right substances to pass into the baby's bloodstream. Your baby receives nourishment through the placenta.

Around the eighth week, your baby will develop eyes (but the lids are still joined together), nose, lips, and tongue. Arms, elbows, forearms, hands, knees, lower legs, and feet begin to form. Before the ninth week, your baby was technically known as an *embryo*. But after the ninth week, it is called a *fetus*. (In this book, we will refer to a fetus as a baby.)

By the end of the first trimester, your baby will be about 3 inches long and weigh about 1½ ounces. The buds and sockets for teeth in the jawbones begin to form. Fingernails and toenails start to develop, the earlobes are formed, and your baby will have most of her or his organs and tissues.

The second trimester   Your baby continues to grow and develop. About a month into the second trimester (4 months) your baby will weigh about 7 ounces and will be 6 to 7 inches long. Your baby's heartbeat will become strong and you may be able to hear it with either your doctor's stethoscope or the doppler device that amplifies the baby's heartbeat. The baby's muscles and bones are formed. Hair grows on the head and eyebrows begin to appear. And you may even feel the baby move!

Near the end of the second trimester (6 months), the baby will weigh close to 1¾ pounds and might be 11 to 14 inches long. You will notice your baby's movements more. The eyelids will separate and eyelashes will form. Also, the fingernails grow to the ends of the baby's fingers.

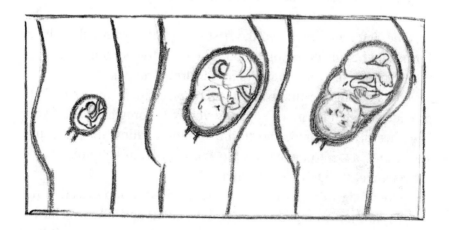

The third trimester   All vital organs are fully formed. The baby's head bones are soft and flexible. Your baby will now begin to gain weight and grow rapidly. By the end of the seventh month, your baby will weigh 2½ to 3 pounds and be 14 to 17 inches long. By the time your baby is ready to be delivered, he or she will weigh about 1¼ to 7½ pounds and be close to 20 inches long.

Diabetes Control and a Healthy Baby

Each of these stages of gestation is important in your baby's development. And it is important that you keep your diabetes in control during each stage. It is *very* important that your diabetes be in control before conception and in the first few weeks of the pregnancy. This is because the baby's vital organs (such as the heart, lungs, kidneys, and brain) are formed in the first eight weeks of gestation. So, a woman must seek care from her health-care team *before* she becomes pregnant.

Babies born to women with diabetes have a higher risk of birth defects than those born to women who don't have diabetes. Researchers suspect that poor diabetes control is responsible for most of these birth defects. Poor control of your diabetes—particularly in those early weeks—could expose your baby to high levels of glucose and ketones. This is because both can pass through the placenta to the baby, but insulin cannot. The baby's exposure to higher than normal levels of glucose may increase the chances for birth defects.

These high levels of glucose can cause other problems for your little one in the last half of your pregnancy. When "fed" this extra glucose, a baby tends to get fat. Because the baby does not have diabetes, his or her pancreas will produce extra insulin to lower the blood glucose. So, the baby grows bigger and fatter than he or she would normally. This condition is called *macrosomia.*

A baby's production of extra insulin can cause another problem. It is hard to quickly stop the baby's pancreas from producing the extra insulin after he or she is born. So, the baby must go through a type of sugar *withdrawal* at birth.

During this withdrawal, the baby's blood glucose level could drop dangerously low, a condition called hypoglycemia (see page 44). If hypoglycemia is not treated, it can cause serious problems for the newborn, such as seizures and cerebral palsy. Usually, the baby is given sugar through an intravenous line (IV) and is watched carefully for several days in the intensive-care unit of the hospital.

Another problem, called *jaundice,* is common among all babies but even more so among those born to women who have diabetes or premature infants. Jaundice is a yellowing of the skin caused from a waste product called bilirubin. Before birth your baby needs a large supply of red blood cells. However, at birth your baby no longer needs this extra supply. So, after the baby is born, its liver will work to break down and excrete the old red blood cells. If your baby's liver isn't mature enough, it may have trouble handling this workload. Unfortunately, this creates a buildup of old red blood cells. The broken-down red blood cells or pigments are *bilirubin.* Instead of being excreted, bilirubin is deposited in the baby's tissues. That is what colors the skin yellow.

Babies born with jaundice are sometimes treated by being exposed to special lights. These lights help break down and get rid of bilirubin. In most children born with jaundice, this treatment is successful and lasts only a few days. But high levels of bilirubin can be toxic to the brain and nerves. If jaundice becomes severe enough, a baby might need a blood exchange, but the chance of this happening is rare.

Another problem that rarely occurs and is not pleasant to discuss is stillbirth. Stillbirth is a word for when a baby dies before birth. Stillbirths used to occur more frequently when women with diabetes had severe hyperglycemia (when blood sugar is too high). But now, with expert care and good diabetes control, the chances for stillbirths are quite low. It may be necessary to deliver the baby a few weeks early to prevent problems, however.

Section 3

Diabetes During Pregnancy

Good diabetes control is important to your good health. And your unborn baby's health depends a lot on how healthy you are. So, good control plays a big role in the health of your unborn baby. If you are planning to have a baby, your diabetes should be in control before you become pregnant. This is because your baby will begin developing as soon as it is conceived—before you even know you are pregnant. And those first several weeks are crucial to your baby's development.

During your pregnancy, your body is going to undergo some drastic changes. Besides changing your appearance, your pregnancy will likely disrupt your diabetes control, which is why you will need to make some changes in your diabetes regimen. You probably will need to alter the amount of insulin and number of injections you take each day, your meal plan, your exercise routine, and the number of times you check your blood sugar each day. Keep in mind that the adjustments you make for the first trimester of your pregnancy may need to be altered for your second and third trimesters. All these changes are designed to keep you and your baby healthy.

Next, we'll discuss the elements that are important to managing your diabetes both before and during your pregnancy.

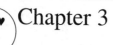

Chapter 3

Insulin Therapy

Diabetes is a disease in which the body does not produce or respond to insulin (a hormone produced by the pancreas.) Without insulin, your body is unable to convert the food you eat into the energy you need to live, work, and play. Your body gets its energy from glucose, a form of sugar that is made from the food you digest. Insulin lowers blood glucose levels by allowing the glucose to enter your body's cells. In other words, insulin acts as a key that unlocks the door to the cells to let glucose in. Only once it is inside those cells can glucose be used for energy. Without insulin, the glucose simply builds up in the bloodstream—a condition that is not healthy for your body.

If you have type 1 diabetes or type 2 diabetes that cannot be controlled by diet, exercise, or diabetes pills, you must inject insulin daily. (Insulin cannot be taken in pill form because your stomach juices would destroy its active materials before they had a chance to work.) Your insulin regimen—the combination of insulins and number of injections you need—will be based on your body's special requirements. As your baby grows, develops, and matures and as you change your schedule and your lifestyle, your insulin regimen will change too.

These changes or adjustments are just one part of the balancing act needed to maintain blood glucose levels as close to normal as possible. "Normal" usually describes the blood glucose levels of a person who does not have diabetes. In these individuals, fasting (or early morning) blood glucose should be under 90 mg/dl. ("Mg/dl" means milligrams of glucose per deciliter of blood—a standard way of measuring blood glucose levels.) About one hour after meals, your blood glucose level should be below 120 mg/dl. (In technical terms, this is called a one-hour post-prandial level or reading.) These are general goals for pregnant women with diabetes; however, your individual blood sugar goals must be worked out with your doctor or health care practitioner.

You will need to make these adjustments in your regimen because once insulin has been injected, it will work according to its action schedule regardless of what you do. In other words, the insulin you injected before breakfast will start lowering your blood glucose level as scheduled even if you didn't get to eat breakfast. So, working with your health care practitioner to find an insulin regimen that suits your body's needs as well as your lifestyle needs is important.

Differences in Insulins

Many people are confused by the variety of available insulins and ask: Is there a difference? The answer is an overwhelming yes. Insulins vary in several ways. Years ago, the only kind of insulin available was animal insulin. Choices included either pork or beef insulin or a combination of the two. Today, synthetic human insulin is used much more often. This human insulin is chemically identical to that produced by a human pancreas, but it is made in the laboratory through a process called genetic engineering. There is also a type of insulin called "insulin analogs." The human insulin is modified to be absorbed faster—lispro and aspart are examples—or slower—glargine is an example.

Insulins also vary in their action times. There are four main types of insulin: rapid acting; short acting; intermediate acting; and long acting. While rapid-acting Humalog (lispro) has not been approved for use in pregnant women, it is prescribed by some doctors because it is very good for maintaining blood glucose control

Types of Insulin

	Form	Peak*	Duration*
Rapid acting (onset less than 15 min)			
Humalog (Lilly)	human	½–1½ h	4–6 h
NovoLog (Novo Nordisk)	human	½–1½ h	3–5 h
Short acting (onset ½–2 h)			
Humulin R (Lilly)	human	2–3 h	6–10 h
Iletin II Regular (Lilly)	pork	2–3 h	6–10 h
Novolin R (Novo Nordisk)	human	2–3 h	6–10 h
Novolin BR (Novo Nordisk)	human	1–3 h	6–10 h
Intermediate acting (onset 2–4 h)			
Humulin L (Lilly)	human	4–12 h	16–20 h
Humulin N (Lilly)	human	4–10 h	14–18 h
Iletin II Lente (Lilly)	pork	4–12 h	16–20 h
Iletin II NPH (Lilly)	pork	4–10 h	14–18 h
Novolin L (Novo Nordisk)	human	4–12 h	16–20 h
Novolin N (Novo Nordisk)	human	4–10 h	14–18 h
Long acting			
Humulin U (onset 6–10 h) (Lilly)	human	10–16 h	20–24 h
Lantus (onset 2–4 h) (Aventis Pharmaceuticals)	human	none	12 h
Mixtures (onset ½–1 h)			
Humulin 50/50 (Lilly)	human	2–12 h	14–18 h
Humulin 70/30 (Lilly)	human	2–12 h	14–18 h
Humalog Mix 75/25 (Lilly)	human	2–12 h	14–18 h
Novolin 70/30 (Novo Nordisk)	human	2–12 h	14–18 h

The time of action of any insulin may vary in different individuals or at different times in the same individual. Because of this variation, the time periods given for the action of insulin should be considered as general guidelines only. See insulin package insert for more information.

and because there is no evidence that it causes harm during pregnancy. Rapid-acting insulins usually reach the bloodstream quickly (often in as little as 5 minutes). This insulin is most effective (meaning that it peaks) about an hour after you inject it. It stays in your bloodstream about 2–4 hours although not at full strength.

Regular, or short acting, insulin usually reaches the bloodstream within 30 minutes, and peaks from 2 to 3 hours after injection. It is effective for about 6–10 hours.

Intermediate-acting insulin takes about 2–4 hours to reach your bloodstream. It peaks 4–12 hours later and can stay in the blood up to 20 hours. Long-acting insulin takes 6–10 hours to reach your bloodstream. These insulins provide a nearly continuous insulin release and are usually effective for 18–24 hours.

While your doctor or health care practitioner will determine the exact combination of insulins you will use, the choice of how many injections you take and the method of insulin delivery depends on how easy it is to control your blood glucose level. Chances are you will need a combination of insulins with different time actions, as well as several injections during the day.

There are several ways you can administer the insulin you need. Today's micro-fine needles make injections relatively painless. Some people choose jet injectors. These are mechanical devices that "shoot" the insulin through your skin in a jet stream. Still, others choose to use insulin pumps. Pumps are small, computerized devices that deliver insulin in a steady drip through a needle under the skin. However, the pump is not recommended for everybody, and you must be highly motivated to use it. Discuss these options with your health care team so that you can make informed decisions.

Insulin and Pregnancy

During your pregnancy, your body will go through some major changes. These changes will affect your blood glucose level and make keeping your diabetes in control difficult. One of the key changes in your diabetes care during pregnancy will be regular adjustments in your insulin program.

As your pregnancy progresses, your need for insulin will increase. This is because during pregnancy, the placenta produces hormones that decrease insulin's ability to lower blood glucose. Some women require double or even triple the amount of insulin

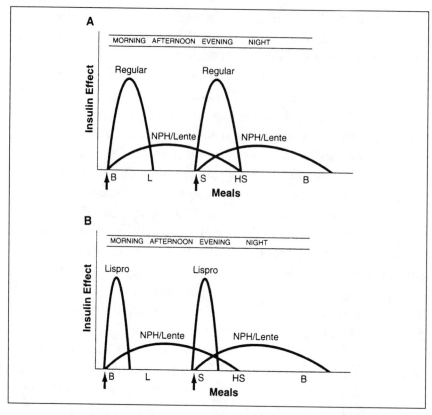

Figure 1 **(A)** Short-acting and intermediate-acting insulin. **(B)** Rapid-acting and intermediate-acting insulin.

they normally inject to maintain the same level of control. So, it's likely you will be put on an intensified insulin program. Like your usual insulin regimen, this intensified program may require that you increase your number of injections to three or four shots a day. The increase in insulin as well as the increase in the number of injections will help your body stay healthy while your baby is developing.

In addition to increasing your insulin program, your blood-testing regimen will probably intensify as well. (See blood glucose monitoring, pages 40–42.) Most women need to make changes in their insulin regimen about every 5 to 10 days because the need for insulin increases rapidly during pregnancy. Before conception and at different stages of your pregnancy, you will probably have a HbA$_{1c}$

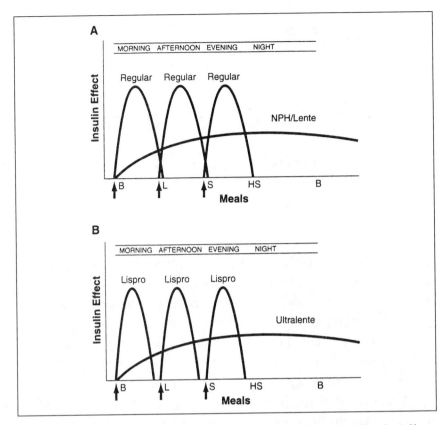

Figure 2   **(A)** Short-acting before meals and long-acting insulin in the morning. **(B)** Rapid-acting with meals and long-acting insulin in the morning.

test (also known as a glycated hemoglobin test). This test is one way to measure your average blood glucose control over the past 2 to 3 months. Along with frequent self-monitoring, this test will help your doctor or health care practitioner adjust your insulin regimen.

If you have questions, don't hesitate to ask a member of your health care team for advice on how to make the necessary adjustments. Ask your physician to teach you to make the necessary changes to keep up with the ever increasing insulin requirements of pregnancy. If you do not have a thorough understanding of insulin adjustments, do not change your own insulin doses. Instead, stay in contact weekly with the health care team to allow

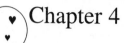

Chapter 4

Nutrition, Diabetes, and Pregnancy

It is almost impossible to achieve good blood glucose control without following a meal plan. This is because food raises your blood glucose level. To keep your diabetes in control, you need to match the carbohydrate in the food you eat with the amount of insulin you inject and the exercise you do. So, it's important to be aware of not only *what* you eat, but also *how much* you eat, *when* you eat it and the grams of carbohydrate in it.

A registered dietitian (RD) or health care professional with nutrition expertise will be able to help you design a meal plan especially for you. Your meal plan should include foods that you prefer and that meet your diabetes needs. Sound awful? Don't jump to conclusions—you may be surprised at how varied and flexible your meal plan can be.

In recent years, some changes have been made in nutrition guidelines for people with diabetes. You are now encouraged to eat more complex carbohydrates, such as vegetables, breads, and pasta; more fiber; and less fat. You may be able to eat small amounts of simple sugars (such as a small piece of unfrosted cake, a cookie, or a small scoop of ice cream) on special occasions—but first check with your RD and doctor to learn how to fit it into your meal plan, and, if necessary, to adjust your insulin dose. While it's true you may not be able to eat as freely as you did before your diabetes developed, you can still eat most foods you enjoy.

Most people with diabetes have three meals a day and several well-timed snacks to make sure there is enough glucose in their blood at the time their insulin is peaking.

You don't have a meal plan? Don't worry. Instead, find a dietitian who can help you design one. If you don't know where to look, ask your health care practitioner for help. Your hospital may also be a good resource. Or the ADA may have a listing of RDs in your area. Call 1-800-DIABETES and ask.

Everyone, with or without diabetes, can benefit from meal planning but this is especially true for mothers-to-be. That's because meal planning is based on the principles of good nutrition. And good nutrition is very important in having a healthy baby. Since it's so important, let's discuss what you need to do to meet the nutritional needs of you and your baby during pregnancy.

Meal Planning for a Healthy Baby

Much like preparing to run a race, you need to get yourself into condition before you become pregnant. Establishing good nutrition and eating habits before your pregnancy is a major part of *getting into condition.* This is true for all women considering pregnancy, but it is especially important for you because you have diabetes.

Of course, you may be more fortunate than many women because you are probably more conscious of what you eat than those who don't have diabetes. In fact, women with diabetes often enter pregnancy with better nutritional habits than nondiabetic women!

Your nutritional needs change during pregnancy for two reasons. First, your baby needs nourishment. Second, your body will change the way it uses certain nutrients. It is important for you to practice good nutrition during pregnancy to fulfill the needs of your baby before birth as well as during lactation (breastfeeding). So let's begin by looking at the nutritional needs of your baby while he or she is developing and growing inside you.

Your Baby's Needs

People once thought that a developing baby could take whatever nourishment it needed from its mother. However, recent research has shown that this theory may not be true. Specifically, the growth and development of a baby is related to the mother's nutritional habits and weight gain. So, losing weight while you're pregnant is not recommended, but eating a well-balanced diet is. Here's why: When a mother doesn't get all the nutrients she needs either because food is scarce or because she chooses not to eat enough, her supply of nutrients for her baby is reduced. The consequences of poor nutrition may include health problems for the mother. It may also result in the birth of an underweight baby with nutritional as well as other deficiencies.

Poor nutrition can also affect the placenta, which does several things that are essential to your baby's health. The placenta transports glucose, amino acids, hormones, and other substances from your body to your baby's system. If you are poorly nourished, the placenta cannot do these things properly.

So, good nutrition throughout pregnancy is important. Part of meeting your nutritional needs is making sure you gain enough weight over the nine months.

Weight Gain During Pregnancy

A weight gain of 22 to 32 pounds is considered appropriate for mothers who are at a normal weight when they become pregnant. Just how much weight you will need to gain is a determination your doctor or health care practitioner will make, based on your body and your baby's needs.

The usual pattern of weight gain is quite small during the first three months—only about 2 to 4 pounds, unless you are underweight. If so, you will need to gain more. As your pregnancy progresses, you will need to gain more to assure adequate fat stores. Fat stores act as a reserve to provide for the added energy needs of you and your baby. In addition, they aid in providing nutrition during lactation. (If you are overweight, less of these fat stores will be needed.)

During the second three-month period, you gain weight at a much faster rate—a little less than a pound a week on average. And during the last three months, the rate in which your body is gaining weight may slow down. Weight gains that follow this pattern have been shown to result in the best outcome of pregnancy. The figure on page 24 shows the different weight gain goals during pregnancy for various groups of women.

During pregnancy, it is more important to consider your pattern of weight gain rather than the total. If you start to gain a lot of weight suddenly or if you stop gaining weight or even start losing weight, your health care team will want to know why. Any unusual changes in your weight should be discussed. If the problem is simply related to the food you eat, talk to your dietitian so that changes can be made in your meal plan.

Weight Gain for Underweight Mothers

About 10% of all women who become pregnant are underweight at the time of pregnancy. Another 10% become underweight because they do not eat properly during pregnancy. It is important to gain the proper weight to reduce the risk of having a baby with a low birth weight. However, there is no proof that forcing yourself to gain weight will also cause your baby to gain weight. So, how much should you gain? The answer is whatever your body needs to ensure a safe pregnancy. Check with your health care practitioner for advice.

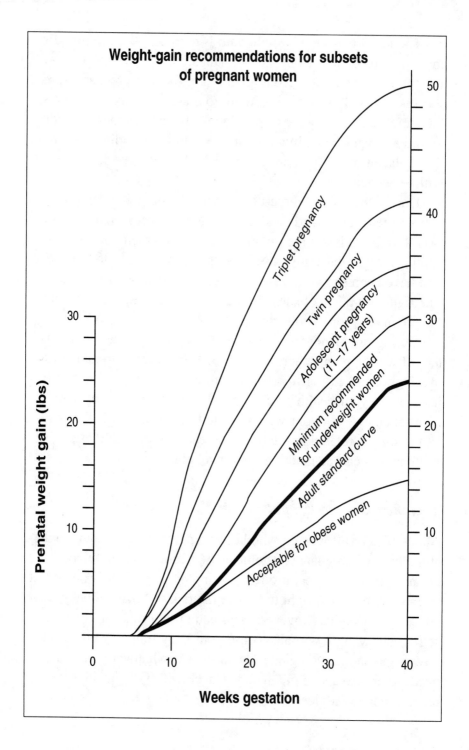

Weight-gain recommendations for subsets of pregnant women

Prenatal weight gain (lbs)

Triplet pregnancy

Twin pregnancy

Adolescent pregnancy (11–17 years)

Minimum recommended for underweight women

Adult standard curve

Acceptable for obese women

Weeks gestation

24

Weight Gain for Overweight Mothers

Mothers who are overweight during pregnancy can also have problems, which may include an increased incidence of *hypertension* (high blood pressure), and *preeclampsia* (hypertension and swelling caused from pregnancy).

If you have had weight problems before pregnancy, what should you know? First, pregnancy is definitely not a time to lose weight. The time to lose weight is before you become pregnant. If you don't eat enough calories during your pregnancy, your system may be forced to burn more fat than usual. This process will produce ketones and is called *starvation ketosis,* which could be harmful to your baby. So weight loss should be avoided (see ketones on pages 48–49).

About 7 to 10 pounds of weight gain during pregnancy comes from an increase in fat stores. If before becoming pregnant you had extra fat stores, you may be able to gain less weight than the lean mother. How much weight you will need to gain will be determined by your doctor or health care professional based on your nutritional needs and those of your unborn baby. In general, if you are obese, weight gain during pregnancy should probably be limited to 15 pounds.

Adolescents and Pregnancy

Teenagers who become pregnant may need to eat more calories than most other women. Because the body of a teenager is still growing, the teen mother needs to provide for her body's own needs as well as for her baby's. Your health care practitioner can help you determine a weight goal.

Distribution of Weight Gain

The following figure shows the average pattern of weight gain and the areas where weight gain occurs. You will notice that during the early part of pregnancy your baby will gain very little weight—not much more than 1 gram (about 1/28 of an ounce) of body weight per day. By contrast, your weight will increase rapidly during this time. Your uterus and breasts will enlarge, your blood volume will expand, and the placenta and amniotic fluid will be formed.

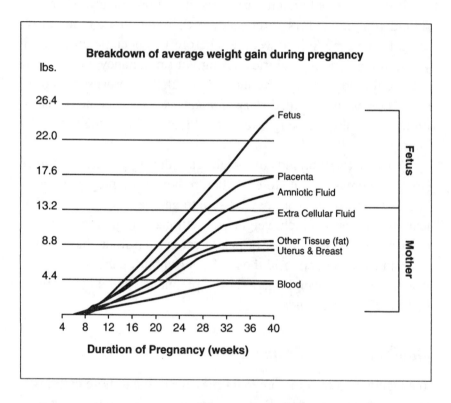

The fat stores in your body will increase rapidly in the early months. Around the fifth month or so, this storage will slow down. One of the first things you may notice when you become pregnant is a gradual thickening of your waist, back, and upper thighs. Don't be alarmed. This is natural and important. Your body is storing nutrients so that some reserves are available to safeguard the nutritional needs of your baby in the following months.

For the first four months, the daily nutrient needs of your baby are very small. However, by the sixth month your baby will gain approximately 10 times the weight each day that he or she gained early in pregnancy.

Calories Needed During Pregnancy

How many calories do you need during pregnancy to meet your weight goals? You need enough to provide your body with the energy it needs to function properly.

The best advice is to work closely with your dietitian to determine your calorie requirements. He or she will, with your help, determine a meal plan for you and your growing baby. Then, by monitoring your weight gain, you and your dietitian will know whether you are getting enough calories.

Nutrient Needs

While you are pregnant, you have some very specific nutrient needs. Your diet should include complex carbohydrates, especially those high in fiber, such as beans and starchy vegetables, whole-grain breads, and fruits. You should also cut down on the fat in your diet. The following are some of the nutrients you need during your pregnancy:

Carbohydrates Most women do well when about 40% of daily calories come from carbohydrates. The best way to ensure you are eating the right amount, however, is to test your glucose levels. Your fasting blood glucose should register 90 mg/dl or less, and one hour after a meal your blood glucose should measure 120 mg/dl or less. ("Mg/dl" means milligrams of glucose per deciliter of blood. It is a standard way of measuring blood glucose levels.)

The recommended carbohydrates are starches, or complex carbohydrates, such as vegetables, beans, pasta, whole grains, tortillas, rice, and wheat breads. In the past, concentrated sweets, such as table sugar, cookies, candy, sodas, jello, fruit juice, and pastries were thought to release glucose rapidly into your blood and cause hyperglycemia (high blood sugar). While there is little scientific evidence to support this theory, these foods should still be avoided. They are high in calories and low in nutrients, and thus can contribute to obesity in the mother-to-be and to macrosomia in her baby.

You may find that counting the carbohydrates in your meal and eating the same number of "carbs" at the same meals from day to day helps you control your blood sugar. It's the carbohydrate in food that raises blood sugar. Watch your serving size.

Fiber   Most fiber is an indigestible form of carbohydrate that is highly recommended for pregnant women. Fiber delays the absorption of nutrients from the intestine and allows the blood sugar to rise gradually after a meal. Fiber also reduces the constipation that often occurs during pregnancy.

Protein   About 20% of your daily calories should come from protein. Good sources for protein are milk and other dairy products, meat, poultry, fish, and legumes (dried beans and peas). During pregnancy, protein helps expand your blood volume and promotes growth of breast and uterine tissues. It is especially important for the growth and development of your baby.

Fat   About 30 to 40% of your daily calories should come from fat. Unfortunately, most people eat too much fat. Fats are high in calories, so they need to be limited. Fat is found in meats, dairy products, snack foods, butter, margarine, peanut butter, salad dressings, oils, and nuts. Be sure to ask your dietitian for tips on how to limit your fat intake to 40% of your daily calories.

Vitamins   Eating a well-balanced diet will usually provide the vitamins and minerals you need while you are pregnant. However, you may not get the amount of iron, calcium, and folic acid you and your baby need. For this reason, your health care practitioner may ask you to take vitamin supplements.

There are two reasons why you need more iron while you are pregnant: to provide for your increase in blood production and to supply iron to your unborn baby, so he or she can produce blood.

Babies store the iron they receive in their livers. If your diet is rich in iron, your baby will be born with enough iron stores to last through the months when he or she is fed mainly milk. (Milk, unless fortified, does not contain iron). Most foods don't contain enough iron for you to get the amount you need during pregnancy. So, unless you are willing to eat liver once or twice a week, you will most likely be asked to take an iron supplement.

You also need more calcium during pregnancy—1200 mg is the recommended daily intake. Calcium is important for bone development and strength. Milk is a good source of calcium. One quart of milk or the equivalent in other milk products (such as four cartons of yogurt) will give you the calcium you need. If you are not able to drink that much milk or if you are allergic to milk, you may need to take a calcium supplement, preferably calcium carbonate. Ask your doctor or dietitian about calcium supplements.

You can get a sufficient amount of calcium by drinking vitamin D-fortified milk, and through exposure of skin to sunlight. Vitamin D is important along with calcium because it promotes calcium absorption.

Another important vitamin to take before conception and during pregnancy is folic acid, which has been shown to prevent certain birth defects. It is common in a variety of foods, but you will likely need to take supplements since you will need almost twice the usual requirement while you're pregnant. Some good sources of folic acid include dark green leafy vegetables (spinach or kale), dried beans, liver, oranges, and whole-wheat products.

The need for other vitamins (such as the B vitamins or vitamin C) increases only slightly during pregnancy. Too much of some vitamins, such as vitamin A, can be harmful to both you and your baby. Therefore, excessive doses should be avoided. Check with your health care practitioner for specific guidelines.

Putting it All Together

You probably still have questions—about artificial sweeteners, alcohol, caffeine and other substances, as well as about when to eat and how much. Some of that information is addressed below, but you should talk with your dietitian or other member of your health care team for guidelines that are specific for you.

Eat small, frequent meals   Eating smaller meals more often during the day can help prevent high blood sugar after meals. Experts recommend three meals and three snacks a day to keep you from becoming overly hungry. Frequent meals can also help you avoid the nausea and heartburn that many pregnant women experience. If you include a protein food with every meal and snack, you'll get double benefits: Protein is digested and absorbed more slowly than carbohydrates, so you will feel satisfied longer and you'll run less risk of hyperglycemia (high blood sugar).

Eat a small breakfast   It is best to avoid fruits and juices and eat a small breakfast of whole grains and protein-rich foods.

Saccharin and Aspartame   Mothers are often concerned about the safety of using artificial sweeteners, such as saccharin and aspartame (Equal or NutraSweet), during pregnancy. Saccharin can cross the placenta to the baby, but no one is sure if this is a problem. So, saccharin should be avoided during pregnancy.

Aspartame is composed of the amino acids aspartate and phenylalanine. Aspartame seems to cause little concern for pregnant women, because these two amino acids are found in most of the protein we eat. It is unlikely that eating or drinking an average amount (such as one can of diet soda or one serving of aspartame-sweetened dessert per day) would be harmful.

Caffeine   Caffeine is a colorless, bitter substance that works as a stimulant, meaning it increases the activity of the heart and central nervous system. It is found in coffee, tea, and many carbonated beverages. In 1981, the U.S. Food and Drug Administration issued a general warning encouraging women to avoid unnecessary caffeine consumption during pregnancy, although an NIH-NICHD study showed that moderate caffeine consumption is safe. So, it's probably a good idea for pregnant women who choose to use caffeine do so in moderation. (Moderation for you may not be the same as moderation for another woman. Ask your health care practitioner how much caffeine is safe for you.)

Alcohol   Today, we know that it can be dangerous to drink alcohol during pregnancy. Women who drink alcohol regularly during pregnancy have a greater risk of delivering a baby with birth defects. Some examples of birth defects are unusual facial characteristics, low birth weight, and defects in the baby's central nervous system that could result in a decrease in intellectual abilities, perhaps even mental retardation.

It appears that low doses of alcohol—such as two glasses of beer a night—if consumed regularly by the mother, may result in growth failure and/or lower IQ in her baby. Even moderate amounts of alcohol seem to double the risk of a miscarriage, as well as growth failure of the baby. No one knows if there is a safe level of alcohol consumption during pregnancy.

The best advice for all pregnant women is to drink no alcohol.

Smoking   Besides being unhealthy for you, cigarette smoking can also be harmful to your baby. Smoking can contribute to having a low birth-weight baby. In contrast to alcohol, most of the growth retardation due to smoking occurs during the last three months of pregnancy. Stopping smoking even as late as the last few months may reduce its harmful effect. Smoking will not affect your weight gain, but it can affect your baby's.

The more a mother smokes, the higher her risk for problems. So, if you can't stop smoking, you should at least try to cut back on the number of cigarettes you smoke. The earlier a mother stops smoking, and the less she smokes, the better.

Cocaine and Other Drugs   While you are pregnant, it is very important that you use only those medications specifically prescribed for you. While so-called "recreational drugs," such as cocaine, are harmful for you at any time, use of these drugs during pregnancy can result in harmful effects for your baby. Some of the problems that can result from using these drugs include birth of an underweight and undersized baby, mental retardation, and abruption of the placenta (premature separation of the placenta from the uterus, a life-threatening condition for the baby). We advise that you totally avoid any harmful drugs during pregnancy.

Nutritional Issues Related to Diabetes

Mothers with insulin-dependent diabetes have additional concerns about nutrition during pregnancy. These include keeping blood glucose within normal ranges during this nine-month period.

To keep blood glucose in line, you will need to stick to your pregnancy meal plan throughout the day. The balancing of food and insulin will help prevent hypoglycemia (low blood glucose, also known as an insulin reaction) and hyperglycemia (high blood glucose).

The importance of eating regular meals and snacks cannot be emphasized enough. Women often respond to an occasional high blood glucose level by skipping a meal or snack, especially at night. However, you need to remember that blood glucose values reflect what has happened during the *previous* one to three hours. When you eat, you are eating to prevent hypoglycemia during the next two to three hours.

If you find that your blood glucose is always high at certain times of the day, call your doctor or health care practitioner to help you make the proper adjustments in your insulin regimen or meal plan.

Bedtime snacks are especially important during pregnancy. Your baby feeds from your supply of glucose 24 hours a day, not just during the hours when you are awake and eating. As a result, overnight low blood sugars are common. Your evening snack should probably include foods containing all three nutrients— protein, carbohydrate, and fat. Milk and other dairy products are a good example. Some women find they even need to eat during the middle of the night. Often, a glass of milk (8 ounces) during the night is enough to prevent the blood glucose from dropping too low. Mothers-to-be also need to check their blood glucose levels during the night, around 3 AM.

During the first three months, you may find you are eating less (and so taking in fewer calories) than you were before you were pregnant. This is especially true if you are nauseated because of morning sickness. As you get over that period, you will probably want to eat more to meet your increasing calorie needs.

How you distribute calories throughout the day is important. Three meals and three snacks are usually recommended. Breakfast is likely to be your smallest meal because blood glucose values are frequently highest in the morning. Blood glucose monitoring can help you and your dietitian schedule your meal plan correctly.

Problems with Pregnancy

Nausea and Vomiting   Try the following for nausea:
- Eat crackers or dry toast when you wake up and before you get out of bed. (Although no research has demonstrated why this helps, it may be related to a low blood glucose level. Remember, these foods are pure carbohydrate, so your morning insulin dose will have to be adjusted to accommodate these foods.)

- Eat smaller meals and eat more often.
- Drink fluids between meals instead of with meals.
- Avoid spicy and greasy foods.
- Avoid lying down right after eating.

Constipation   Constipation is common during pregnancy. One reason is because your intestinal muscles become more relaxed. Another reason is that your growing baby puts more pressure on your intestines. If you have problems, try the following:
- Drink plenty of water or caffeine-free noncarbonated liquids.
- Eat high-fiber foods, including whole-grain breads, bran cereal, raw fruits, and vegetables.
- Get plenty of exercise.
- If the problem persists, discuss it with your health care practitioner.

Heartburn   As your pregnancy progresses, you may get heartburn. Some symptoms of heartburn include burning discomfort in the stomach or throat, an upset stomach, or a stomachache. The following may help:
- Eat frequent, small meals.
- Avoid greasy or spicy foods.
- Eat slowly, being sure to chew food well.
- If heartburn persists, check with your doctor for help.

Cravings   At some stage in pregnancy many women find that their food likes and dislikes change. During their pregnancy, some women may dislike foods they normally like. At the same time, they may have a craving for foods they normally would not eat. So, you may need to make changes in your meal plan to fit your new likes and dislikes. Your dietitian will work with you.

Medications   Since many medications can be harmful to your baby, avoid all medications except those prescribed for you during your pregnancy. Check with your doctor before using any over-the-counter medications.

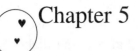

Chapter 5

Exercise, Diabetes, and Pregnancy

Physical activity is good for you, especially when you have diabetes. In most cases, exercise will lower your blood glucose
level. Exercise is also helpful in losing weight, which is a concern
for many people who have diabetes. (Caution: Do not attempt to
lose weight while you are pregnant unless you are under a health
professional's care.) Exercise can also help improve your muscle
tone, circulation, and heart function. Finally, exercise is beneficial
because it can give you a feeling of well-being.

All women are unique, and some are more fit than others.
Some are able to run marathons, while others have conditions that
prevent them from doing any strenuous exercise. So, it is important to find a level of exercise that's safe for you before, during,
and after pregnancy. Exercise can be beneficial, but only when it is
done correctly and at a safe level. Be sure to discuss an exercise
program with your doctor before you start. Your doctor needs to
check the condition of such things as your eyes, blood pressure,
and heart. These checkups are important to be sure you are physi-
cally ready to exercise and to see whether your body can handle an
exercise program as it adjusts to the stress of pregnancy. When you
become pregnant, you should discuss any changes that may need
to be made in your exercise program as your pregnancy progresses.

Finding a good exercise program is not the only thing. Besides the struggle you may have getting the ambition to exercise, you need to think about how your exercise will affect your diabetes. In most cases, exercise lowers blood glucose. Therefore, whenever you exercise, it is important to monitor your blood glucose level. This means checking your blood before and after you exercise. If your blood glucose level is 200 mg/dl or above, you should not exercise. When your glucose level is this high, exercise may only raise it higher. And when you are pregnant, if your blood glucose level reaches 240 mg/dl, you should contact your physician immediately. (Ideally, you should already know what to do if your blood glucose is this high. Usually you take a few units of rapid-acting insulin immediately.) Remember that exercise can affect your blood glucose levels for up to 24 hours after you've stopped exercising.

Monitoring your diabetes also means learning to recognize the symptoms of low blood glucose or hypoglycemia (see page 44) during and after you exercise. To help avoid hypoglycemia, it is important to coordinate your exercise program with your meals and with the timing and amount of insulin you inject. If you exercise more (or less) than you planned or at a different time, you may upset your blood glucose level. Your health care team will be able to help you work your exercise program into your diabetes regimen.

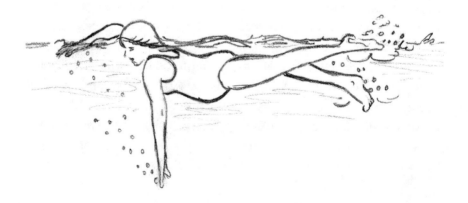

If you feel low blood sugar coming on while you are exercising, stop and treat it with some form of sugar. You can use 4 ounces of orange juice, 2 or 3 pieces of hard candy, 4 ounces of a nondiet soft drink, or 3 glucose tablets. Your dietition may have some other suggestions. Once you feel better, you should eat some protein, such as half a meat sandwich, a piece of cheese, or a glass of milk.

By working closely with your health care team, carefully monitoring blood glucose, balancing food and insulin, and exercising at an appropriate level, you are doing all you can to maintain good diabetes control. Be smart and take the time to prepare properly for any exercise routine. Also, be careful not to overdo it—too much exercise too soon can be harmful for anyone.

Exercise and Pregnancy

You may already be a part of a growing number of women who are regularly involved in exercise programs. Like many of these women, you may have concerns about whether you can continue your exercise routine after you become pregnant. And because you have diabetes, you likely have questions about how exercise will affect your blood glucose control during pregnancy.

In the past, pregnant women with diabetes were advised not to exercise because many people feared exercise would affect the health of the baby. Today, however, women who have regularly exercised before pregnancy can often continue exercising during pregnancy. Of course, they may need to exercise at a more moderate level while they are pregnant. If you have not been involved in regular exercise, you should not start a strenuous exercise program while you are pregnant. Whether you have been exercising or not, there may be some exercises that you won't be able to do during this time.

Exercises you may need to postpone include such things as racquet sports, golf, volleyball, and basketball. These activities involve twists, turns, jumping, and sudden starts and stops—all of which can strain your muscles, joints, and ligaments and may have a harmful effect on your baby. You should also avoid hazardous activities such as water and snow skiing. (The potential harm is falling at high speeds.) Many women should also avoid jogging while pregnant. (Falling is a concern, but the pounding could prove harmful to your pregnancy.)

While you may have to postpone some activities, there are other exercises you can do to stay fit. For example, brisk walking may be a good alternative. Many people who found jogging too strenuous have benefited from walking. A brisk walk after a meal may be ideal for controlling your diabetes. This may be especially true after breakfast, since many times blood glucose levels are highest in the morning.

Swimming can also be good exercise for many women who are pregnant. It isn't bone-jarring or hard on your feet and legs and the buoyancy of the water eases stress on your joints. Thus, you are freer from injuries. Some communities or local YMCAs offer water aerobics classes.

You may also be able to participate in an aerobics program, but at a lower level than you may be used to. A good alternative may be low-impact aerobics. This method allows you to get an aerobic workout but is designed to lessen the impact on your body.

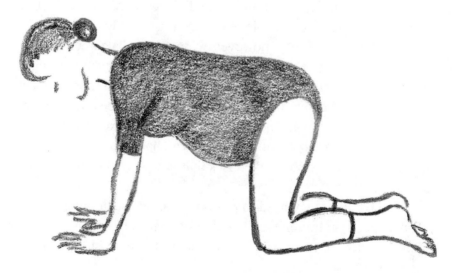

Tai chi or yoga for pregnant women are low-impact exercises that can help you strengthen your muscles while you gain or maintain flexibility. They contribute beneficial stress relief, too. But if you've never done yoga before, don't start a "regular" class after you become pregnant. Find one for pregnant women.

Another safe form of exercise is to sit in a sturdy chair with good back support and lift 1- or 2-pound weights. Push the small of your back against the chair; *never* arch your back to lift a weight.

Postnatal Exercises

Remember, your need for fitness never stops—not even during the excitement of caring for your baby and rescheduling your life to meet your baby's needs. Exercising after the birth of your baby is essential to good diabetes control. It will also help your body make the major adjustments after pregnancy. Toning your muscles helps your body get back to the firm shape it was before you were pregnant. If you don't exercise, you may find it much harder to tighten your body up later.

You can probably start exercising soon after your baby is born. If you have a cesarean section, you may have to wait a little longer. Ask your health care practitioner when you can safely return to your prepregnancy exercise program or start your new one.

Chapter 6

Monitoring Your Diabetes

To know how well you are controlling your diabetes, you have to test your blood and your urine. These tests will help you make the needed adjustments to keep your diabetes control on target. This chapter explains blood glucose monitoring and urine tests and the role each plays in your diabetes control.

Blood Glucose Monitoring

In the early 1980s, self-monitoring of blood glucose became available. This advance has made it possible for you to test your blood glucose anywhere you choose. Self monitoring has contributed greatly to diabetes management and has increased your chances of having a successful pregnancy as well.

Of course, if you check your blood but fail to make needed adjustments in your diabetes regimen, blood testing won't do you any good. It is important that you record the results of each check so that you and your health care team can see how well your diabetes regimen is working. Your record will show if you need to make changes.

There are two ways to test your blood. In both, you first prick your finger with a special needle called a lancet to get a drop of blood. You then place the drop of blood on a test strip. The steps you follow to do your blood test will depend on what method you use to read the test strip. Ask your doctor or health care practitioner to talk you through the testing process you need to follow.

In one method, you wait for the test strip to change colors. (The glucose causes the change.) You then match the color of the strip to a color chart, which is usually on the test strip container. The colors represent *ranges* of glucose levels, such as 60 to 90 mg/dl. If your test strip colors match those colors, then your blood glucose level falls somewhere in that range. You only use this method if you don't have your meter or it's not working correctly.

In the second method, you place the test strip in a blood glucose meter. A meter is a small computerized machine that reads your test strip and displays your blood glucose level on a digital screen (like that of a pocket calculator).

Meters provide more accurate blood glucose readings than matching the test strip colors to a chart. This is because meters give you an exact number instead of an estimate or range of your blood glucose level. And as you prepare for pregnancy or if you are pregnant, accuracy is extremely important. A meter is essential.

Most people with diabetes are now advised to check their blood glucose four times a day as a way of tracking diabetes control. Generally, tests are done before breakfast, lunch, and dinner, and at

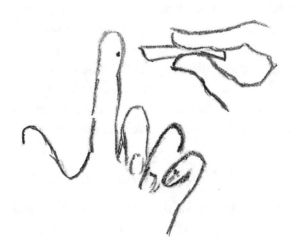

bedtime. During your pregnancy, you may be asked to check after your meals or even during the night. Blood checks, like insulin therapy, are individually tailored to each woman and her pregnancy.

Urine Tests

Before blood glucose monitoring became available, urine tests were the only way a person could monitor diabetes control. But now, because of the accuracy of blood glucose testing, urine tests are no longer used to monitor diabetes control. That's because urine tests can only give you an estimate of your glucose level. In fact, the reading from a urine test may actually show what your glucose level was hours before the test rather than what it actually is at the moment of testing. Such an estimate will not provide you with the information you need to maintain good or tight diabetes control.

Still, urine tests do provide vital information that will help you detect *ketoacidosis*. In fact, testing your urine is the only way to measure ketones (see ketones, page 48). Ketones are bad for your health and that of your baby. While you are pregnant, you are at a higher risk for developing ketones because pregnancy increases your metabolic rate. So, you may be asked to test your urine for ketones more than you did before you were pregnant.

Urine tests are fairly easy to do. First, you take a sample of your urine and place a test strip in the sample. Like the blood glucose strips, this strip will change color. You match the color to a chart, which will give you an indication or range of the amount of ketones present in your urine. If your urine test detects ketones, you should contact your health care practitioner.

Making Adjustments

As you work to control your diabetes, it's likely you'll need to make adjustments occasionally—some major ones, some minor ones. You may have to change your meal plan, your exercise routine, or insulin dosage—or possibly all three—because of the changes your body undergoes during pregnancy. For example, most women need to make changes in their insulin regimen about every 5 to 10 days because the need for insulin increases rapidly during pregnancy.

Other things may make it necessary for you to make adjustments. For example, you may change jobs, have a different work schedule, or become more active. Sometimes you have to make sudden adjustments because of changes in your daily routine, such as an unexpected physical activity. Sometimes your diabetes regimen is just not working to control your diabetes.

The important thing to remember is not to feel you are stuck with a certain diabetes program. If you are having trouble controlling your diabetes, adjustments will need to be made. Members of your health care team can help you set up guidelines for changing your diabetes regimen when needed. You should never make changes without first checking with your doctor or health care practitioner.

Recording the results of your blood glucose checks and urine tests is important because this information is vital to making adjustments in your diabetes regimen. You may need to record how much carbohydrate is in your meals and snacks. There is a direct relation between the amount of carbohydrate you eat and the insulin you need to take. As you and your health care team work together, you should be able to find an insulin regimen that will work to keep you healthy.

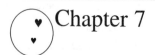

Chapter 7

Problems Associated
with Diabetes

It would be wonderful if practicing good diabetes control could eliminate all the difficulties that relate to diabetes. Unfortunately, it just isn't so. While you have a better chance of preventing any problems by adhering to your diabetes regimen, you will still experience occasional problems with such things as hypoglycemia, hyperglycemia, and ketones. The trick is detecting these problems early and treating them before they get worse. If left untreated, these problems can have serious consequences for you and your baby. That's why we've chosen to discuss each in more detail.

Hypoglycemia

Hypoglycemia is low blood sugar. It is sometimes called an insulin reaction. Hypoglycemia can be caused by a number of things: You may have taken too large a dose of insulin, eaten too little food, not eaten on time, or exercised too much.

Testing your blood is the best way to know whether your blood glucose is low. But there are other symptoms that will help ᴐu recognize low blood sugar. The symptoms include:

- shakiness or dizziness
- sweating
- ᴉumsy or jerky movements

44

- hunger
- headache
- sudden moodiness or behavior changes, such as crying for no apparent reason
- pale skin color
- difficulty paying attention or confusion
- tingling sensations around the mouth

If you experience any of these symptoms, eat some quick-acting sugar. Then check your blood sugar. If you can't test, you should treat the reaction. It is better to have too much sugar than to suffer severe low blood sugar.

You can treat hypoglycemia by eating or drinking some form of sugar. Some examples are 3 to 4 pieces of hard candy or sugar cubes, 4 ounces of orange juice, 4 ounces of a regular (nondiet) cola drink, or 3 glucose tablets. About 20 minutes after you treat an insulin reaction, you should check again just to be sure your blood glucose level has risen. If it hasn't, you may need to eat more. After you feel better, eat some protein, such as a couple pieces of cheese, half a sandwich, or 8 ounces of milk. Low blood sugars should always be recorded in a notebook because your health care team needs to know about them.

Note: These are only suggestions. You should check with your dietitian for specific ways to treat low blood sugar during your pregnancy.

Hypoglycemia is always a potential problem for a person with diabetes, but it can be particularly so during pregnancy. This is because hypoglycemia can occur more rapidly and without the usual warning signs. To avoid problems, we recommend checking blood glucose when insulin is peaking, or most effective. For example, if you inject regular insulin at 7:30 AM and eat your normal meal as scheduled, your insulin would be most effective about three hours later. So, you would want to check your blood glucose level between 10 and 10:30 AM If your blood glucose level was below 60 mg/dl, you would most likely increase your morning snack according to the instructions of

Warning Signs of Hypoglycemia

- shakiness or dizziness
- sweating
- clumsy movements
- hunger
- headache
- sudden moodiness or behavior changes, such as crying
- pale skin color
- difficulty paying attention or confusion
- tingling sensations around the mouth

your health care practitioner, or decrease your morning insulin dose.

You should always be prepared to treat hypoglycemia, but especially when you're pregnant. To be safe, you should have a glucagon kit in your home and at work for severe cases of hypoglycemia. Glucagon is a hormone that causes your blood sugar to rise. It is used primarily to treat someone who has passed out from hypoglycemia. It is a good idea to teach family members and co-workers how and when to inject glucagon, just in case a severe reaction should happen to you. A member of your health care team can write you a prescription and teach you how to use glucagon.

Hyperglycemia

Another problem that accompanies diabetes is *hyperglycemia.* Hyperglycemia is high blood sugar. It happens when your body has too little insulin or when too much food is eaten.

Hyperglycemia can happen for several reasons. You may eat more than you planned or exercise less than planned. Other things can cause hyperglycemia, such as the stress of an illness like a cold or the flu. Emotional stresses, such as family or work conflicts, may also contribute to hyperglycemia. The signs and symptoms of hyperglycemia include:

- high levels of sugar in the urine
- frequent urination

- increased thirst
- headaches
- tiredness and fatigue

Like hypoglycemia, the best way to avoid hyperglycemia is to test your blood regularly and then treat high blood sugar early before other symptoms appear. Your doctor can tell you what level is considered high. Generally a blood glucose level of 120 mg/dl or above is considered high during pregnancy.

If you do not treat hyperglycemia, a condition called keto-acidosis (diabetic coma) could occur. Ketoacidosis happens when your body has too many ketones (see ketones, page 48). Ketoacidosis needs immediate treatment because it is life-threatening.

How do you treat hyperglycemia? There are three ways to lower blood glucose levels—exercise, eat less food, take more insulin. The method you use will depend on the circumstances at the time of the high blood glucose reading. You and your health care practitioners need to work out procedures for handling one-time instances of hyperglycemia as well as more detailed instructions for handling patterns of high blood sugars.

Exercise is often the first method used to lower blood glucose. If this does not work, you may be asked to eat less at a given meal or snack. Finally, you may have to change the amount of insulin you inject or the timing of the injections. Your practitioners should be able to help you find the best way to lower your blood glucose.

You should not change your diabetes regimen without first checking with your health care team. (If you are pregnant and your blood glucose tops 240 mg/dl, call your health care practitioner for immediate help. Blood glucose levels this high may be harmful to your baby.)

How will hyperglycemia affect your health or the health of your baby while you are pregnant? If your diabetes is not in control during the early part of your pregnancy, you increase the risk of having a baby with birth defects.

Signs and Symptoms of Hyperglycemia

- high blood sugar
- high levels of sugar in the urine
- frequent urination
- increased thirst
- headaches
- tiredness and fatigue

Hyperglycemia also increases the chance of having a large baby who may go through a "sugar withdrawal" at birth. In a sense, your baby may become addicted to your high blood sugar. This means that once the baby is born, he or she may become severely hypoglycemic because the level of blood sugar is not as high as he or she was getting inside of you. This condition could cause the baby to have seizures. Also, a large baby increases the risk that you will have your baby by cesarean section (see page 58).

Testing for Ketones

Ketones are acid substances that are produced when the body breaks down fats because no other source of energy is available. This process happens when there is not enough insulin to let glucose (the main source of energy) enter the cells and provide the body with the energy it needs. Your body cannot tolerate large amounts of ketones and will try to get rid of them through the urine. Unfortunately, your body cannot get rid of all the ketones, so they build up in your blood.

Small amounts of ketones in the morning are not uncommon during pregnancy. Check with your doctor for the specifics of how you should handle this condition. You should test your urine for ketones whenever your blood glucose is greater than 200 mg/dl (see urine testing, page 42). Ask when and how often you should test for ketones, especially while you are pregnant.

If ketones continue to build up in the blood, a condition called ketoacidosis could happen. Ketoacidosis can be life-threatening and needs immediate treatment. It is different from hypoglycemia in that it usually develops gradually over many hours. There are several warning signs of ketoacidosis:

- a dry mouth
- thirst (but not hunger)
- nausea
- excessive urination
- dry skin
- fruity-smelling breath
- abdominal pain
- vomiting
- if advanced, unconsciousness

Whenever you detect any of these symptoms, you should contact your health care practitioner. Usually, ketoacidosis must be treated in the hospital, where fluids can be restored and diabetes can be brought under control.

Warning Signs of Ketoacidosis

- a dry mouth
- thirst (but not hunger)
- nausea
- excessive urination
- dry skin
- fruity-smelling breath
- abdominal pain
- vomiting
- unconsciousness, if advanced

More about Pregnancy

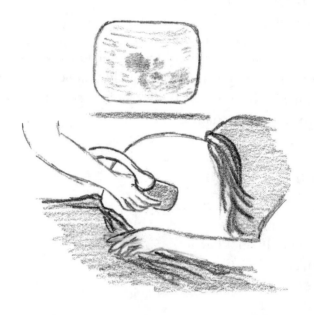

Labor and delivery—finally, the moment arrives when all the work you have done to keep you and your baby healthy pays off. For most women, the birth of their baby is an exhilarating, joyful experience. Of course, labor itself is not fun, and it is natural for you to be a little scared or apprehensive about delivering your baby. However, because of the technology available to monitor your health and that of your baby, the chances for a successful pregnancy are now better than ever.

So, relax. Take a deep breath. Let it out slowly. Turn the page and focus your thoughts on the next chapters.

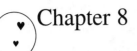 Chapter 8

Tests to Expect During Your Pregnancy

During your pregnancy, you will probably go through several different types of tests, technically known as *antepartum* testing. (Antepartum means before labor or childbirth.)

In general, antepartum testing is divided into two categories. In the first category are those tests given during the first half of pregnancy, called *diagnostic prenatal testing*. These tests are intended to detect structural or genetic disorders in your developing baby.

The second category of tests is started later in pregnancy, usually in the third trimester, and are often continued until delivery. These tests are called *fetal surveillance*. Some of these tests measure your baby's growth. Others evaluate the condition of your baby. This is done by checking how well the placenta supplies your baby with oxygen and nutrients. Here are tests that you may experience during your pregnancy:

Diagnostic Prenatal Testing

Serum Alpha Fetoprotein (AFP)   During the first part of the second trimester (around 16 weeks from your last menstrual period), an AFP test may be ordered. This test measures the level of AFP in your blood and looks for neural tube defects such as spina bifida or anencephaly. (The neural tube is the initial organ from which your baby's brain and spinal cord develop. Spina bifida is a defect in the spinal cord. With anencephaly the brain does not develop fully.) The risk for these defects is quite low. Among women with diabetes, only 6 to 8 per 1,000 will have a baby with neural tube defects, and serum AFP testing will identify 75% of these pregnancies.

The AFP test is a *screening* test that identifies those pregnancies that are at risk; it does not make a specific diagnosis. In other words, this test tells you something is not right, but it cannot tell exactly what is wrong. Many factors other than a neural tube defect can cause the AFP level to be abnormal. In fact, 5 of each 100 women tested will have an abnormal test value. When this happens, other diagnostic procedures, such as ultrasound or amniocentesis, are used. Many women whose test results show abnormal values go on to deliver perfectly healthy babies.

Diagnostic Prenatal Testing

- Serum Alpha Fetoprotein (AFP)
- Ultrasound
- Genetic Counseling and Testing

Ultrasound   Ultrasound tests use sound waves to outline and photograph organs—including a developing baby—inside the human body. The picture that is taken is called a *sonogram*. This procedure has been used for decades, and studies have not revealed any harmful effects to mothers or their babies.

Before the test, you may be asked to drink lots of fluids. So that your bladder will be full, you will also be asked not to urinate. This allows the person doing the test to make certain measurements more easily. (There is also a way to check the baby using a vaginal probe; this does not require the woman to have a full bladder.)

The procedure uses a machine with a monitor screen to produce the pictures. The testing is painless. You lie on your back while a moveable arm or probe (called a *transducer*) is gently glided across your abdomen. Ultrasound testing identifies the number of babies, their position in the uterus, and the outline and structure of their bodies. Ultrasound is usually performed in the second half of pregnancy. By this time, the baby is large enough for all the distinct features to show up on the test. It can sometimes detect the sex of your baby, though sex determinations are not always accurate. It also helps in estimating how far along your pregnancy is. However, it is not always possible to identify birth defects with a sonogram.

There is one piece of evidence that suggests that an ultrasound performed at eight weeks of gestation may identify birth defects. When the fetus is too small at this age, there is a 30% risk of a defect.

Because you have diabetes, your baby may be larger or smaller than average. Ultrasound is often repeated at monthly intervals to determine your baby's rate of growth.

Genetic counseling and testing   Just because you have diabetes does not mean you are automatically more at a risk for giving birth to a baby with genetic disorders. However, other factors unrelated to diabetes may present an increased risk for genetic problems in your baby. For example, when the mother is 35 years or older, the risk of genetic disorders increases. A previous family history of genetic disorders is also a factor. Some common genetic disorders are cystic fibrosis, muscular dystrophy, and Down's syndrome.

If you are at risk for having a baby with genetic disorders, you may be referred for genetic counseling. This includes an evaluation and explanation of your specific risk for delivering a child with a particular genetic disorder. Testing options, including the risks of the procedures, will be explained.

The most common type of genetic testing is a procedure called *amniocentesis,* which is usually done around the fourth month of pregnancy. It is performed by taking a sample of the amniotic fluid that surrounds the baby (the bag of waters).

When amniocentesis is performed, ultrasound is used to find the baby and the best "pocket" of fluid. A needle is then inserted through the mother's abdomen to remove a small amount (usually less than an ounce) of the fluid, which is then tested in a laboratory to make a diagnosis. Most of the time, this test is done by growing some of the cells (a tissue culture) that were floating around in the fluid. Growing the tissue culture takes weeks. Experts then examine the tissue culture to determine the genetic structure.

Waiting for these test results—and knowing the results themselves—may be emotionally difficult for you and your partner. The decisions you and your partner may have to make as a result of these tests could also be difficult. For this reason, you should receive as much information as possible about your particular risks and the options available to you.

Some decisions you make about yourself and your family are very difficult, but *only you* can make them. Being informed is vital. Your health care team is available to provide emotional support when you need it.

Fetal Surveillance

A number of methods to evaluate the health of a developing baby have been devised over the years. No method is clearly superior to the others—different centers caring for high-risk pregnancies vary in their choice of tests. It is best to use the test (or tests) that a particular center is most familiar and comfortable with. This is fine since all methods are designed to provide similar information about your developing baby's health.

Fetal Surveillance

- Kick Count
- Non-Stress Test (NST)
- Biophysical Profile (BPP)
- Amniocentesis

The commonly used tests are described here; you may receive one or more of them.

Kick counts   The movements or kicks that you feel from your baby are one important indicator of your baby's health. You may be asked to count the number of times you feel your baby move during a particular time each day. Your doctor or nurse-educator will explain how and when to do these counts. He or she will also explain how to recognize serious problems and when to alert your health care practitioner. In general, when you detect a change in the pattern of your baby's movement, you should notify your health care team. They may want to do further testing.

Non-Stress Test (NST)   This test determines the state of your baby and the placenta by measuring changes in your baby's heart rate when he or she kicks. A fetal monitor placed on your abdomen checks the acceleration (speeding up) of your baby's heart rate at times of activity. This acceleration suggests that your baby is healthy. The test is painless and usually takes 30 to 45 minutes and can be performed in your doctor's office.

Biophysical Profile (BPP)   In this test, ultrasound is used to evaluate your baby's movement, body tone, breathing, and the amount of amniotic fluid surrounding your baby. (Although there is no air in your uterus, your baby does make breathing motions while inside you. Amniotic fluid is drawn in and out of the lungs.)

Amniocentesis   This procedure was discussed on pages 53–54 under diagnostic prenatal testing; however, it is also useful in fetal surveillance. Amniocentesis helps determine when it is safe to deliver your baby. Sometimes it is necessary to induce labor or deliver a baby by cesarean section (see page 57). Before either procedure is performed, it may be necessary to find out whether your baby's lungs are mature. If your baby is delivered before the lungs are mature, a problem called *respiratory distress syndrome* may make it difficult for your newborn to breathe normally. By doing amniocentesis to obtain amniotic fluid, a test can be done to see if your baby's lungs are mature enough to breathe on their own. This test will help predict whether respiratory distress syndrome is likely. The actual procedure is exactly the same as that described earlier, but the results of the test are usually available within 24 hours.

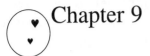

Chapter 9

Labor and Delivery

Before we knew the techniques for tight control of blood glucose, the risks for giving birth to a very large baby or for having a stillbirth were quite high. In the past, a woman with diabetes was usually admitted to the hospital during the final weeks of pregnancy and delivery was induced early.

Now that self-monitoring of blood glucose is possible, most women with diabetes can remain safely at home until labor begins. And they can have their babies on or near their due dates. Hence, fewer premature babies are born to women who have diabetes. (Premature babies may have immature lungs and have trouble breathing after delivery.)

After studying your health and that of your baby and how your pregnancy is progressing, your health care team will determine the best time and mode of delivery for both you and your baby. It's possible that your labor will start on its own and your baby will be born vaginally (through the vagina). If your labor does not start on its own, it may be induced with a hormone called pitocin. Pitocin speeds up labor by causing the uterine muscles to contract. If you can't deliver your baby vaginally or if there is a problem, then you will need to have your baby by an operation called a cesarean section (C-section) or cesarean birth.

During a C-section, an incision is made through the abdomen and uterus, through which the baby is removed. Because of the surgery, your recovery may be longer than if you delivered your baby vaginally. Generally, a woman who has a C-section needs to stay in the hospital 4 to 5 days and takes 4 to 6 weeks to fully recover.

Many babies born to women with diabetes are delivered by a C-section. The reason may be because many give birth to large babies who cannot fit through the birth canal.

However, the size of your baby is not the only reason a C-section may be necessary. In some cases, labor can be stressful for a baby, and a C-section may be necessary to ensure the baby's health. If you've had a C-section before, you may choose to deliver future babies this way. Finally, health complications may make a C-section necessary. Be sure to discuss a C-section with your health care team months before your baby is born. It's best for you to be prepared for whatever may happen.

To determine the safest time and method to deliver your baby, your health care team will examine a variety of factors: blood glucose control, blood pressure, kidney function, and diabetes complications. The team will also study your baby's size and movements, his or her heart-rate pattern, and the amount of amniotic fluid in the uterus.

In some cases, a small amount of fluid will be withdrawn from your uterus (see amniocentesis, page 53). This procedure will help determine whether your baby's lungs are mature and help guide the timing of delivery. While you are in labor, your baby's heart rate and well-being will probably be tracked by a fetal monitor.

Keeping your blood glucose level as normal as possible will be a major concern during your labor and delivery, regardless of when or how your baby is delivered. Your having a normal glucose level during labor and delivery will reduce the risk of your baby having low blood glucose after delivery. Remember, if your blood glucose is high, the glucose crosses the placenta and may cause your baby's pancreas to produce too much insulin.

Labor, like any strenuous exercise, tends to lower blood glucose in a person whose diabetes is well controlled. So, you will probably need less insulin during active labor. Your blood glucose will be checked frequently (probably every few hours) and your insulin and glucose regimen will be tailored to your needs during this time. You may want to take your blood glucose testing equipment to the hospital with you. In some hospitals it will take much longer for the nurse to get the equipment than it will for you to do your own blood glucose check.

It's obvious that you want to be prepared by knowing what you can about your pregnancy and the birth of your baby. That you're reading this book demonstrates your interest. To help you prepare for labor, many hospitals and other organizations offer classes (such as Lamaze) to help you have a smooth delivery. They teach you what to expect during labor, techniques to improve delivery and to relieve pain during labor, and how to care for your baby after birth. If you're interested in such a class, ask your doctor or check with your hospital about classes in your area.

Finally, we want to add this warning: Some women desire to give birth in the home. Because of the care needed to perform a successful delivery, home births are not recommended for women who have diabetes.

Lactation

Nearly all women are encouraged to breastfeed their babies. Breast milk is healthy for the baby: It contains antibodies to fight certain infections. Breast milk has other advantages, too—it is readily available, inexpensive, and convenient. In addition, breastfeeding will help you bond with your baby. Breastfeeding can also help you lose some of the weight you gained during pregnancy. It might even prove a good way to help you lose any excess fat you had before you were pregnant.

In addition, there is increasing evidence that breastfeeding your infant for at least 3–6 months may help protect your baby from developing diabetes in the future.

Most women lose between 12 and 15 pounds during the first week after giving birth. The total weight you gained during pregnancy should be gradually lost over a 3-month period. If your health care practitioner recommends that you lose weight, you can begin during the time you are breastfeeding. However, you should generally wait two to four weeks after your baby's birth before you begin to lose this weight.

During the time that you breastfeed, you need to pay close attention to what you eat. The meal plan you had before you were pregnant may not cover the demands of breastfeeding. If you are in doubt, check with your dietitian to find a meal plan to meet your needs.

While you are breastfeeding, it is important that you get the right amounts of calcium, fluids, and protein. Breast milk is amazingly constant in composition, but the quantity of milk changes depending on how much fluid you drink. If you reduce the amount of food that you eat, the quantity of your milk will also be reduced. You and your dietitian can discuss and plan your meals to fit your needs while you are breastfeeding.

Breastfeeding may also require insulin adjustments, especially in your overnight dosage. This is because your blood glucose level may drop quickly while you are breastfeeding especially during your baby's bedtime and late-night feedings. Ask how to make these adjustments and whether you need to add a snack or two.

While breastfeeding may be a perfect way to nourish your baby, you may be unable or unwilling to breastfeed. Some women are uncomfortable breastfeeding. Some have full-time jobs that make breastfeeding on a regular schedule difficult. Others, because of health reasons, are unable to breastfeed. If you can't or don't want to breastfeed, don't feel guilty. Your baby can still do well and get the nutrients he or she needs from a formula. And it's important to note that there are soy-based formulas that do not contain cow milk products. Using these formulas may protect the child from developing diabetes in the future in much the same way as breast milk.

After Delivery
(The Postpartum Period)

Soon after you give birth, major changes will occur. Your weight and level of activity will change during this time. Also, you may experience emotional ups and downs—many new mothers do. After your baby is born, your insulin needs will be much less than they were during your pregnancy.

For a short time, your insulin needs may even be less than they were before you became pregnant. Blood glucose monitoring is the best way to chart these rapid changes and will make it easier to make the necessary adjustments as your body returns to its nonpregnant state. A few weeks after delivery, your insulin dose should return to the level it was before you became pregnant.

If you didn't take control of your diabetes before you were pregnant, you probably learned a great deal from taking control during your pregnancy. Now that you're in the habit, it will be easier to continue practicing good control. You'll be happy you did—and so will your new family.

Section 5

Birth Control

Birth Control
The Pill
Diaphragm
Condom
Intrauterine Device (IUD)
Rhythm Method or Sympto-thermal Method
Depo-Provera Injections
Norplant system
Sterilization

Some women may wonder what a section on birth control is doing in a book about pregnancy. Many of you may think it's a little late to be talking about that now. However, there are a couple of reasons for this section. First, this book is not just for the woman who is pregnant, but also for the woman who is *thinking* about having a baby. She needs to consider birth control until she is ready to have a baby. Second, after a woman has a baby, birth control is important.

There are many options on the market today and it is important that you and your partner consider each one. Some methods of birth control may work better and fit into your lifestyle more easily. Some are safer for you than others. Making an informed choice, which includes discussing birth control with your doctor, will help increase the chances of choosing a method with a high success rate, and one with fewer health risks to you.

Chapter 10

Making the Choice

Choosing the safest and most appropriate time to have a child is one of the keys to planning a successful pregnancy for a woman with diabetes. Of course, *planning* a pregnancy means that you are going to use some form of birth control (contraception) until you are ready to try to have a baby.

Many women with diabetes are concerned about the safety of various methods of contraception, the advantages and disadvantages of each, and whether one method is better than the others. One of the most important aspects of family planning is choosing the right method of birth control for *you* and your partner.

A number of different methods are available and no one method is right for *all* individuals. You have special needs that may make one form of birth control better for you than another. The important factor in choosing any method is that it should be reliable and effective. Unfortunately, not all the methods available today offer the protection you need. It is important that you and your partner discuss and find a birth control method that suits both of you. Here are some of the birth control methods being used today:

The Pill   Oral contraception, or the birth control pill, is one of the most popular methods of birth control. However, popularity doesn't mean the pill is the best choice for you. The advantage of birth control pills is their reliability. They are 99% effective *when taken as directed.*

The "pill" refers to a variety of oral contraceptives made from synthetic forms of two hormones involved with regulating the menstrual cycle, estrogen and progesterone. The synthetic form of progesterone is called progestin. A combination estrogen and progestin pill is slightly more effective than progestin alone (99% as compared to 98% success rate). The progestin-only pill can also cause irregular bleeding and weight gain.

In some instances, even today with lower dosage pills, taking oral contraceptives can worsen blood sugar control. If this is the case, your diabetes treatment program may need to be adjusted accordingly, or you and your partner will have to agree on other options. Second, the pill may put a woman at risk for heart disease or stroke. The pill can cause a rise in blood fat levels (cholesterol, LDL, and triglyceride levels). It can also cause problems with circulation and clotting. But as the dose of estrogen and progestin has been decreased in newer pills, so has the risk decreased for these problems.

However, the risk for circulation and clotting problems is still quite high for women who smoke. Smoking causes the blood vessels to narrow, the walls of the vessels thicken, and the blood to clot. That's why it is important for a woman to quit or reduce her smoking as much as possible. High HbA_{1c} levels may also increase the chances of having blood-clotting problems.

If you choose to take oral contraceptives, it is important to have your HbA_{1c}, blood fats, and blood pressure checked before and routinely after starting the pill. If you have high blood pressure or high blood fats (hyperlipidemia), you may need to use a different method of contraception. Taking the pill when you have high blood pressure can increase the chance that eye or kidney disease will get worse. If you are concerned, speak to your doctor.

Side effects from the pill, such as weight gain, irritability, breast pain, or break-through bleeding are more common with progestin-only pills. If you experience any discomfort with taking any oral contraceptive, it is important to discuss other options with your health care provider. For the best results, keep your diabetes under reasonable control, take the pill as prescribed, and inform your health care provider when you have side effects.

Diaphragm   The diaphragm is a rubber cap that the woman lubricates with a spermicidal gel and fits into her vagina and over her cervix before intercourse. It acts as a barrier to prevent sperm from entering the uterus. The uterus is where eggs are fertilized by the sperm. For this reason, the diaphragm is called a *barrier method* of birth control. When used correctly, it can be up to 95% effective in preventing pregnancy.

Some women find a diaphragm awkward and difficult to use. And they fear it affects the spontaneity of lovemaking. Because the diaphragm can be inserted as much as an hour before intercourse, however, a little planning ahead will allow you to have some level of spontaneity. If you choose a diaphragm, it is important that your doctor fit it properly. Also, make sure he or she explains how to use it correctly. When women with diabetes use the diaphragm, they may have more yeast infections than woman without diabetes.

Condom   Another barrier method of birth control is the condom, a thin membrane sheath that fits over the penis. There are larger ones made for women that cover the outer labia and fit into the vagina. A condom can be used effectively by itself, but it is even more effective when combined with a sperm-killing foam or vaginal gel. Statistics show that when the condom and foam are used together, they are up to 85% effective in preventing pregnancy. The major problem with barrier methods of birth control, such as the condom, is that they require some planning for use. They must be used every time intercourse occurs, and they must be used correctly. If not, they won't be effective. Condoms also protect against sexually transmitted diseases (STDs).

Intrauterine Device (IUD)   An IUD is a small plastic device that is placed inside the uterus by a physician. It works by irritating the uterine wall, which makes it difficult for a fertilized egg to become implanted. In the past, some IUDs were suspected to cause pelvic infections or trauma to the uterine wall, but the newer IUDs are considered to be far less likely to do so. The IUD may be an attractive option for the woman who is not likely to have any more children and has a single sex partner (it does not protect against STDs). It is also an effective choice for women with diabetes because it does not affect blood glucose and blood fat levels. You should discuss with your doctor or health care provider any benefits or risks involved in your using an IUD.

Rhythm Method   The oldest but by far the least effective method of birth control is the rhythm method. In general, it works by avoiding intercourse or using a barrier method during a woman's fertile phase—about 6 to 7 days before ovulation and 2 to 3 days after. For this method to work, you have to know exactly when you ovulate. Most women ovulate during the middle of their menstrual cycle. But cycles can be irregular so it can be difficult to pinpoint the exact time of ovulation.

The best, yet still inaccurate, method of determining when you ovulate is to measure your temperature. This is because body temperature rises slightly at the time of ovulation and remains elevated until your next period. To be as accurate as possible, you need to check your temperature *daily* in the early morning *before* you get out of bed. Since it is possible for pregnancy to occur 6 days before this rise in temperature, you must be diligent in measuring and recording your temperature patterns. You should not rely on this method if you have irregular periods or irregular body temperature patterns. The rhythm method does not protect against STDs.

Depo-Provera   An injection of a progesterone-like hormone that prevents pregnancy for 12 weeks. This method has the advantage of being safely used while breastfeeding (starting 6 weeks after delivery). However, you may not be able to become pregnant for a full year after you stop using Depo-Provera.

Norplant System   This system is not recommended for women with diabetes.

Sterilization   Either female tubal ligation ("tying the tubes") or male vasectomy. Both are simple surgical procedures that are permanent methods of sterilization. Neither affect sexual desire or ability.

Finally, while we are on the subject of birth control, you may wonder how soon after giving birth you can have intercourse. Unfortunately, there are no absolute answers to this important question. It is probably a good idea to wait at least 3 or 4 weeks to give the muscles in the walls of your vagina time to strengthen. And if you had an episiotomy, it will need time to heal. (An episiotomy is an incision made between the vagina and anus to help keep that area from tearing during the vaginal birth of your baby.) Check with your doctor to see how long he or she suggests you wait.

Also, remember that you could become pregnant soon after you give birth. Even if you have not had a menstrual period, you still may ovulate. Also, breastfeeding your baby will *not* prevent you from becoming pregnant.

Choosing birth control is a personal matter—the decision is up to you. But be sure to discuss the different types of birth control with your health care provider. The more information you have, the more likely you will make the decision that will be best for you.

Conclusion

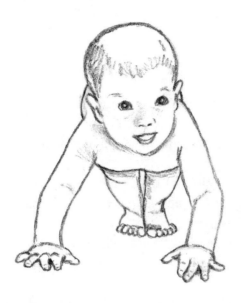

As you can see, the success of your pregnancy depends a lot on how well you take control of your diabetes. At first, controlling your diabetes during pregnancy may seem impossible. It is normal for you to feel that way, but you can do it! True, it will take time and it will take dedication. The important thing to remember is that your health care team will help you make the adjustments you need to keep your diabetes in control during this very special time.

Of course, the most important thing to remember is the end result—a happy, healthy, beautiful baby. Once that baby is born, we're sure you'll agree that the time you took to control your diabetes was well worth it!

Glossary

Abruption (ablatio placentae): Separation of the placenta from the uterus while the fetus is in utero. It can be life-threatening for the baby and requires emergency medical treatment.

Amniocentesis: Puncture of the amniotic sac (bag of waters) with a needle to obtain a sample of fluid for examination.

Bilirubin: The broken-down red blood cells or pigments deposited in the baby's tissues, indicating jaundice.

Carbohydrate: A class of food that raises blood glucose once it is digested.

Endocrinologist: A physician who specializes in glandular diseases. Diabetes is a disease of the gland called the pancreas.

Gestational Diabetes (GDM): Diabetes that occurs during pregnancy and goes away after pregnancy. GDM is diagnosed based on a standard glucose tolerance test.

Glucose: A simple sugar.

Hyperbilirubinemia: Elevation of bilirubin above normal.

Diabetes & Pregnancy: What to Expect ♥

Hyperglycemia: Blood glucose levels above normal. If left untreated, can lead to coma and death.

Hypoglycemia: Blood glucose levels below normal, which can result in sweating, irritability, shakiness, a fast pulse, or unconsciousness if not corrected.

Insulin: The hormone necessary to help the body use and/or store glucose.

Ketosis: Breakdown of body fat into acids that occurs when the body does not have enough food or enough insulin.

Lethargic: Very sleepy.

Neonatologist: A pediatrician who specializes in caring for newborn infants.

Non-stress Test (NST): Monitoring of the baby's heart rate (pulse) when he or she kicks.

Obstetrician: A physician who specializes in caring for pregnant women.

Oxytocin: The hormone that causes the womb to contract.

Pancreas: The organ in the body that produces the hormone insulin.

Pediatrician: A physician who specializes in caring for children.

Placenta: The organ between mother and baby that allows nutrients and glucose from the mother to be passed freely into the baby's bloodstream, but does not allow insulin to pass.

Prematurity: Birth before the baby is mature.

Sonogram: A sound wave picture of the baby.

Stillbirth: The death of an unborn child. Technically this term is reserved for unborn children more than halfway along in the womb.

Registered Dietitian (RD): Also known as a Nutritionist. A specialist in food and meal planning.

Uterus: Womb.

Index

Conception
diabetes control prior to, 11
Condom, 66
Constipation, 28, 34
Contraception, 62–68
Cravings, 34
Cystic fibrosis, 52

D

Delivery, 56–58
Dentist, 7
Depo-Provera, 67–68
Diabetic coma. See
Ketoacidosis
Diabetologist, 5, 6
Diagnostic prenatal testing,
51–54
Diaphragm, 66
Dietitian, 5, 6–7, 20, 45
Down's syndrome, 53
Drug use, 34. See also
Medications

E

Eating habits. See Meal plan;
Nutrition
Embryo, 9
Endocrinologist, 7
Evening snack, 32
Exercise
adjustments to routine, 37,
43
blood glucose level and,
36, 47
postnatal, 39

during pregnancy, 37–38,
58
safe level, 35
Eye doctor, 7

F

Fat, 28
Fat stores, 26
Fetal alcohol syndrome, 31
Fetal monitor, 55, 58
Fetal surveillance, 51–52,
54–56
Fetus, 9
Fiber, 28
Folic acid, 29
Food cravings, 34

G

Genetic counseling and
testing, 53–54
Glossary, 70–72
Glucagon kit, 46
Glucose. See also Blood
glucose level; Blood
glucose monitoring,
baby's exposure to,
11–12

H

Health care team, 5–8, 43
Heartburn, 33
Hemoglobin A_{1c} test, 19, 65
Home births, 59
Hyperglycemia, 58
prevention, 46

symptoms, 47
treatment, 46–47
Hypertension, overweight
mothers, 25
Hypoglycemia
in newborn baby, 12
prevention, 32, 45
symptoms, 44–45
treatment, 36, 45

I

Insulin injections
frequency, 19
methods, 15
Insulin pumps, 17
Insulin reaction. See
Hypoglycemia
Insulin regimen adjustments,
14–19, 33, 43, 45, 47,
59
Insulins
animal vs. human, 15
estimated action times, 16
intermediate-acting (NPH
or lente), 17
long-acting (ultralente), 17
rapid-acting, 15, 17
regular or short-acting, 15
types of, 16
Intercourse after birth, 68
Intrauterine device (IUD), 67
Iron, 29

J

Jaundice in newborn baby, 12

Jogging, 38

K

Ketoacidosis (diabetic coma)
detection, 42
treatment, 48–49
warning signs, 49
Ketones
baby's exposure to, 12
urine test for, 42, 48
weight loss and, 25
Kick counts, 54–55

L

Labor, 57–59
Lactation, 59–60
Lamaze classes, 59

M

Macrosomia, 11
Meal plan
adjustments to, 30, 42
need for, 20–22
while breastfeeding, 58–59
Medications, 34. See also
Drug use
Milk
breast milk, 60
consumption during
pregnancy, 29
Minerals, 29
Morning sickness, 33
Muscular dystrophy, 53

N

Nausea, 33

Neonatologist, 5
Non-stress test (NST), 55
Norplant system, 68
Nurse-clinician, 5
Nurse-practitioner, 5, 6
Nutrient needs, 27–32
Nutrition, 20–32

O

Obstetrician, 3, 5, 6

P

Pediatrician, 5
Phenylalanine, 29
Physician, 5
Pitocin, 57
Placenta, 9, 22
Planned pregnancy
    methods, 61–67
    necessity of, 4, 13
Podiatrist, 7
Postpartum period, insulin
    needs, 60
Preeclampsia, overweight
    mothers, 25
Progesterone, 65
Protein
    after insulin reaction, 37
    in diet, 28
Psychologist, 7

R

Registered dietitian (RD), 5,
    6–7, 20, 44

Respiratory distress syndrome,
    55
Rhythm method, 67

S

Saccharin, 30
Serum alpha fetoprotein (AFP)
    test, 51–52
Sexually transmitted diseases
    (STDs), 66
Skiing, 38
Smoking, 31, 65
Social worker, 7
Sodium, 30
Sonograms, 52
Spina bifida, 51–52
Stages of development
    first trimester, 9–10
    second trimester, 10
    third trimester, 10
Starvation ketosis, 25
Sterilization, 68
Stillbirth, 12, 57
Sugar withdrawal at birth, 11,
    48
Swimming, 38

T

Tai chi, 38
Tea, 31
Teenage mothers, 25
Testing. See Blood glucose
    monitoring; Urine
    tests; names of specific
    tests

Tests. See Antepartum testing
Trimesters, 9

(U)

Ultrasound tests, 52
Urine tests
  accuracy, 42
  recording results, 42
Uterus, 26, 57, 58

(V)

Vitamin supplements, 29
Vomiting, 33

(W)

Walking, 38

Water aerobics, 38
Weight gain
  distribution of, 23–26
  goals, 22–23
  overweight mothers, 25
  pattern of, 22–24
  underweight mothers, 23
Weight loss
  after delivery, 60
  during pregnancy, 25
Weights, 39

(Y)

Yoga, 38

About the American Diabetes Association

The American Diabetes Association is the nation's leading voluntary health organization supporting diabetes research, information, and advocacy. Its mission is to prevent and cure diabetes and to improve the lives of all people affected by diabetes. The American Diabetes Association is the leading publisher of comprehensive diabetes information. Its huge library of practical and authoritative books for people with diabetes covers every aspect of self-care—cooking and nutrition, fitness, weight control, medications, complications, emotional issues, and general self-care.

To order American Diabetes Association books: Call 1-800-232-6733. http://store.diabetes.org [Note: there is no need to use **www** when typing this particular Web address]

To join the American Diabetes Association: Call 1-800-806-7801. www.diabetes.org/membership

For more information about diabetes or ADA programs and services: Call 1-800-342-2383. E-mail: Customerservice@diabetes.org www.diabetes.org

To locate an ADA/NCQA Recognized Provider of quality diabetes care in your area: Call 1-703-549-1500 ext. 2202. www.diabetes.org/recognition/Physicians/ListAll.asp

To find an ADA Recognized Education Program in your area: Call 1-888-232-0822. www.diabetes.org/recognition/education.asp

To join the fight to increase funding for diabetes research, end discrimination, and improve insurance coverage: Call 1-800-342-2383. www.diabetes.org/advocacy

To find out how you can get involved with the programs in your community: Call 1-800-342-2383. See below for program Web addresses.

- *American Diabetes Month:* Educational activities aimed at those diagnosed with diabetes—month of November. www.diabetes.org/ADM
- *American Diabetes Alert:* Annual public awareness campaign to find the undiagnosed—held the fourth Tuesday in March. www.diabetes.org/alert
- *The Diabetes Assistance & Resources Program (DAR):* diabetes awareness program targeted to the Latino community. www.diabetes.org/DAR
- *African American Program:* diabetes awareness program targeted to the African American community. www.diabetes.org/africanamerican
- *Awakening the Spirit: Pathways to Diabetes Prevention & Control:* diabetes awareness program targeted to the Native American community. www.diabetes.org/awakening

To find out about an important research project regarding type 2 diabetes: www.diabetes.org/ada/research.asp

To obtain information on making a planned gift or charitable bequest: Call 1-888-700-7029. www.diabetes.org/ada/plan.asp

To make a donation or memorial contribution: Call 1-800-342-2383. www.diabetes.org/ada/cont.asp